Salt of the Heart

The Devastating Effects of Too Much Salt on Human Health

ALICE HART

Table of Contents

Introduction

The human heart is one of the most important organs in the body, and its health is closely linked to salt intake. Too much salt in the diet can have adverse effects on the heart and lead to an increased risk of heart disease, stroke, and other cardiovascular problems. In this book, we will discuss the effects of salt on the human heart and how to maintain a healthy salt balance in order to protect the heart.

We will also look at the risks associated with consuming too much salt, as well as tips on how to reduce salt intake in order to maintain heart health. Finally, we will consider the potential benefits of salt and how it can be used as part of a healthy diet. By understanding the effects of salt on the human heart, we can make informed decisions about our dietary habits and maintain a healthy balance of salt intake.

Chapter one

Contamination of salt

Salt has been a part of the human diet for centuries, and it is an important nutrient for the body. However, in recent years, salt has become increasingly contaminated with a variety of pollutants. These pollutants include heavy metals, pesticides, and other chemicals that can be hazardous to human health. Heavy metals, such as lead, mercury, and arsenic, can be present in salt due to runoff from industrial sites, mining operations, and agricultural activities. Long-term exposure to these metals can cause health problems, including anemia, kidney damage, and neurological issues. In extreme cases, heavy metal poisoning can lead to death.

Pesticides are another common contaminant of salt. These chemicals are used to protect crops from pests, but they can also enter the environment and contaminate salt. Pesticides can cause various health problems suchPesticides can cause various health problems such as headaches, nausea, and respiratory issues. They can also damage the immune system and can be particularly dangerous to children and pregnant women.

Other chemicals, such as nitrates and chlorides, can also be found in salt. These can come from industrial waste, fertilizers, and sewage. Consuming high levels of these chemicals can cause a variety of health problems, including headaches, nausea, and breathing difficulties. Overall, the contamination of salt with a variety of pollutants is a serious issue.

It is important for people to be aware of the potential health risks associated with consuming contaminated salt. It is also important to take steps to reduce the amount of salt contamination, such as using water filters, avoiding the use of certain industrial products, and buying salt from reputable sources.

Chapter two

Negative health effect of excess salt intake

Consuming too much salt can have a number of negative impacts on our health. Excess salt intake has been linked to hypertension, stroke, heart disease, and kidney disease. This is because when we consume too much salt, our body retains more water, causing an increase in blood pressure. This can damage the blood vessels and increase our risk for cardiovascular disease.The most recent data we have been given is that consuming an excess of salt in out diet can give you ulcers, as per new exploration did, it has been found to assist with sustaining the microscopic organisms behind most stomach ulcers, prompting side effects going from gentle consuming sensations to really retching blood.

Large numbers of these cases are brought about by the Heliobacter pylori bacterium, which fools the stomach into the over creation of corrosive substances consequently causing ulcers and medical affliction. Analysts observed that elevated degrees of salt are causing hereditary changes in this bug making it even more resistant, and cautioned that we ought to all find out about the wellbeing gambles related with an excessive amount of salt.

The food Principles Organization suggests that grown-ups ought to eat something like 6g of salt, which is identical to around 2.5g of sodium. For kids, clearly it fluctuates with age.

Normally, parents shouldn't add salt to youngsters' food and most certainly not to children as their kidneys can't deal with elevated degrees of it, and as a matter of fact it has been known that a lot of it has been deadly in kids younger than one.

We are becoming mindful that for good wellbeing we ought to know precisely exact thing salt we are devouring in our eating routine, yet it is troublesome today to realize exactly how much as an ever increasing number of individuals today eat processed dinners and ready made food varieties, and these items don't necessarily in all cases have clear and exact amounts shown.

Food makers are adding sodium to many sorts of food that we couldn't have ever envisioned contained it, or of the amount, on the grounds that evidently our range 'taste buds' have changed throughout the long term saying that shoppers anticipate this 'taste' now. Our taste buds are for the most part a decent manual for how salty our food is, yet producers likewise regularly use sugars in these food sources that camouflage the saltiness and boneheads our taste buds

Specialists presently say that for the most part just 6% of salt is really added to food at the table, 9% added while cooking and an incredible 75 % of all what we devour comes from ready made food and this includes bread, puddings and breakfast cereals.

Wellbeing experts have been lobbying for clear marking of the amount utilized in the assembling of food sources and for more noteworthy consciousness of the wellbeing worries with eating a lot of salt.

Additionally, too much salt can contribute to weight gain, as our bodies have difficulty processing and excreting the sodium. This can lead to both obesity and an increased risk for diabetes. In addition to physical health concerns, eating too much salt can also have psychological effects on our mental health. Excess salt intake has been linked to irritability, anxiety, and depression. This is because sodium can act as a stimulant and can interfere with our bodies' natural production of serotonin a hormone associated with mood regulation. Overall, it is important to be mindful of our salt intake to maintain our physical and mental health. Eating a balanced diet with adequate fruits and vegetables and limiting the amount of processed foods can help us maintain a healthy sodium intake. Finally, it is important to be aware that some individuals may be more sensitive to the effects of excess salt intake, such as pregnant women, those with hypertension, and those with kidney disease. It is important to consult with a doctor or nutritionist to determine the best diet for each individual. By taking the time to understand our own bodies and the effects of dietary salt, we can make sure we stay healthy and happy.

Chapter three

How to Reduce Salt Intake

Reducing salt intake is a critical part of maintaining a healthy lifestyle. It is important to understand the effects of consuming too much salt and be aware of how to make changes in your diet to limit your intake. First and foremost, it is important to read labels and be mindful of the amount of salt in processed and packaged foods. Many of these foods contain large amounts of sodium, and it is important to be aware of what you are eating. Look for foods that are low in sodium, or are labeled "reduced sodium" or "no salt added." It is also important to limit the amount of salt you add to your food. Try to only season with herbs and spices instead of salt, and avoid adding salt to your cooking water.

You can also reduce the amount of salt you use in recipes by cutting the amount in half and gradually reducing it further. When eating out, try to choose dishes that are made with fresh ingredients and are not pre-salted or pre-seasoned. Ask for sauces and dressings on the side so that you can control how much salt you add. Finally, it is important to be mindful of hidden sources of salt such as bread, cured meats, and canned vegetables. Try to opt for fresh, unprocessed options as much as possible.

By following these steps and being mindful of your salt intake, you can take an important step towards maintaining a healthy lifestyle.

By making small changes to your diet and being mindful of your salt intake, you can easily begin to reduce the amount of salt in your diet and improve your health.

Chapter four

How to recognise and treat high blood pressure

High blood pressure, also known as hypertension, is a condition in which the force of the blood pushing against the walls of the arteries is too high. It can lead to serious health problems such as stroke, heart attack, and kidney disease. Recognizing and treating high blood pressure is essential for maintaining good health.

The first step in recognizing and treating high blood pressure is to understand the symptoms. Common signs and symptoms include headaches, dizziness, chest pain, shortness of breath, and blurred vision. It is important to keep track of any changes in your blood pressure, especially if you experience any of these symptoms. The next step is to visit your doctor for a check-up. Your doctor will measure your blood pressure, perform a physical exam, and review your medical history. Based on this information, your doctor can diagnose high blood pressure and recommend a treatment plan.

Treatment options for high blood pressure include lifestyle modifications such as exercising regularly, eating a healthy diet, reducing stress, and quitting smoking. In addition, your doctor may prescribe medications such as ACE inhibitors, beta-blockers, and diuretics. It is also important to monitor your blood pressure at home. Home blood pressure monitors are available for purchase and are easy to use.

Regularly monitoring your blood pressure and taking your medications as prescribed by your doctor can help to keep your blood pressure under control. Recognizing and treating high blood pressure is essential for maintaining good health. Taking the steps outlined above can help you to manage your blood pressure and reduce your risk of serious health complications.

Chapter five

Healthy alternative to salt

Fortunately, there are many healthy alternatives to salt that can help you to reduce your sodium intake without sacrificing flavor. First, you can use herbs and spices to add flavor to your meals. Parsley, basil, oregano, rosemary, thyme, and other herbs are a great way to add flavor without the added salt. You can also experiment with different dried spices such as garlic powder, onion powder, cumin, paprika, and chili powder. Second, you can try adding acidic ingredients such as lemon juice, lime juice, or vinegar to your dishes. These can add a pleasant tart flavor as well as providing a boost of nutrition. Third, you can use condiments such as salsa, mustard, and hot sauce to add flavor to your meals.These condiments are often lower in sodium than traditional table salt and they can give your dishes an extra kick of flavor. Fourth, you can experiment with reducing the amount of salt you use in your recipes. Start by reducing the amount of salt by half, and then gradually reduce the amount until you find the flavor you like.

Finally, you can use natural sweeteners such as honey and maple syrup to add a hint of sweetness to your dishes. This can help to reduce the amount of salt you use, while still

providing a pleasant sweetness.

Chapter six

Five recipes of low sodium heart friendly foods

1. Grilled Salmon with herbs

Ingredients: - 4 salmon fillets

- 4 tablespoons olive oil

- 2 tablespoons fresh chopped herbs (such as oregano, thyme, and parsley)

- Salt and pepper to taste

Instructions:

1. Preheat the grill to medium-high heat.

2. Place the salmon fillets on a large plate.

3. Drizzle the olive oil over the salmon and season with the herbs, salt, and pepper.

4. Grill the salmon for 4-5 minutes per side, or until it flakes easily with a fork.

2. Baked Fish with Lemon and Garlic

Ingredients:

- 4 fish fillets

- 2 tablespoons olive oil

- 2 garlic cloves, minced

-Juice of 1 lemon

- Salt and pepper to taste

Instructions:

1. Preheat the oven to 375°F.

2. Place the fish fillets in a baking dish.

3. Drizzle the olive oil over the fish and sprinkle

with the garlic, lemon juice, salt, and pepper.

4. Bake for 10-15 minutes, or until the fish

3. Quinoa with Roasted Vegetables

Ingredients:

- 1 cup quinoa, cooked

- 1 cup mixed vegetables (such as broccoli, bell peppers, and carrots), chopped

- 2 tablespoons olive oil

- 2 tablespoons fresh herbs (such as oregano, thyme, and parsley), chopped

- Salt and pepper to taste

Instructions:

1. Preheat the oven to 375°F.

2. Place the vegetables in a baking dish.

3. Drizzle the olive oil over the vegetables and season with the herbs, salt, and pepper.

4. Roast for 20-25 minutes, or until the vegetables are tender.

5. Serve the roasted vegetables over the cooked quinoa.

4.Paleo Taco Salad

Ingredients:

Creamy spicy dressing

-2 ounces hemp seeds (1/2 cup) raw, soaked for at least 4 hours

-2 tbsp olive oil (extra virgin)

-2 tbsp water (filtered or spring)

-1 tbsp white vinegar use lemon juice if not on the migraine diet

-1 clove garlic

-1/2 tsp white pepper

-1/2 tsp smoked paprika (pimenton)

-1/2 tsp cumin (dried)

-1 sprig Italian flat-leaf parsley (fresh) or cilantro

-4 small cherry tomatoes

Taco seasoning:

-2 tbsp chili powder preferably California chili powder

-2 tbsp smoked paprika (pimenton)

-1 tbsp cumin (dried)

-1 tbsp garlic powder

-1 tbsp onion powder (omit for migraine diet)

-1/2 tsp oregano (dried)

-1/4 tsp chipotle powder or cayenne

Salad:

-16 ounces beef (grass-fed) ground (see above for vegan substitutes)

-2 bell peppers (capsicum), red and yellow, thinly sliced

-2 onions (green) scallions, spring onions, sliced on the diagonal

-4 cups romaine lettuce salad greens, spring mix

-1 pint cherry tomatoes

-1 avocado

-3 radishes thinly sliced, or jicama cut into sticks

Instructions:

Creamy spicy dressing

1.Soak the hemp seeds in filtered water for at least four hours. Drain and rinse thoroughly.

2.Place all dressing ingredients in the blender and blend until smooth and creamy. Set aside.

Taco seasoning

1.Mix all ingredients together until one color. This makes enough for two recipes.

Salad

1.Heat a cast-iron skillet over medium-high heat. Add the beef, breaking up with a spoon and cooking until no longer pink.

2.Sprinkle 3 tbsp taco seasoning evenly over the beef and add one cup (200 ml) of filtered water. Stir to mix thoroughly. Continue to cook over medium heat until the moisture is gone and beef is cooked. Remove beef to a warm plate. Do not wipe out the pan.

3.Add 1 tbsp (15 ml) coconut oil, extra-virgin olive oil, or rendered bacon fat to the pan, tilting to coat evenly.

4.Sauté the peppers and the green onion for 10 minutes until golden and fairly limp.

5.To serve, lay out ingredients on a large platter with the dressing on the side.

5.mushroom stew

Ingredients:

-1 tbsp rapeseed oil

-1 clove garlic, peeled and crushed

-2 shallots, peeled and thinly sliced

-2 celery stalks, trimmed and sliced

-250g (9oz) closed cup mushrooms, sliced

-1 tsp paprika

-3 tbsp red wine (optional)

-7fl oz passata

-1 low-salt vegetable stock cube

- 7oz potatoes, peeled and diced

-4½oz canned butterbeans (drained weight – equivalent to a small 210g can)

-1oz low-fat soft cheese

-Small pinch garlic granules (optional)

-1 tbsp fresh parsley, chopped

Instructions:

1. Heat the oil in a pan and fry the garlic, shallots, celery and mushrooms for five minutes until they begin to soften. Sprinkle over the

paprika and stir well. Add the passata, and wine if using. Crumble in the stock cube, along with 200ml boiling water. Stir, reduce the heat and cover. Simmer for 20 minutes.

2. Meanwhile, bring a pan of water to the boil and cook the potatoes until tender – this will take about 15 minutes. Then add the canned butterbeans to the pan of water and cook for two to three minutes more so they heat through. Drain well and mash with the soft cheese, and garlic granules if using.

3. Serve the stew with the butterbean mash and sprinkle with chopped parsley. (If freezing, allow the stew to cool and place into a freezer-proof container, putting the mash in a separate

container. Defrost both overnight in the fridge, then reheat in covered dishes for 20 minutes at 200°C/180°C fan/gas mark 6.)

Conclusion

In conclusion, it is clear that too much salt in the diet can have devastating effects on human health. From an increased risk of hypertension to dehydration, salt can cause serious physical and mental health problems. Therefore, it is important to be aware of the amount of salt in our diets and to try to reduce it as much as possible. With a healthier diet and lifestyle, we can all enjoy the benefits of a low-salt diet. Salt is essential for life, but too much can be dangerous. With a well-balanced diet and proper hydration, we can ensure that we are getting the necessary amount of salt without overdoing it.

By following these guidelines, we can enjoy the benefits of a healthy and delicious diet without having to worry about the risks associated with excessive salt intake. Salt is an important part of our diet, and it can also be a tasty addition to many dishes. However, it's important to remember that too much salt can be dangerous, and can have long-term health implications. By being aware of the effects of excessive salt on our bodies, we can make sure to enjoy the salt of the heart without any major health risks.